Transformative Whirling

Shahram Shiva's Unique & Proven 4-Step Method to Whirling

by
Shahram Shiva

Rumi Network
www.Rumi.net

Publication
Title: Transformative Whirling
Subtitle: Shahram Shiva's Unique & Proven 4-Step
Method to Whirling
Written by: Shahram Shiva
Published by: Rumi Network
Year of Publication: 2018
ISBN: 9781976892561
Number of Pages: 58
© Copyright Shahram Shiva
All Rights Reserved.

Websites
www.Rumi.net
www.ShahramShiva.com

Social Media
www.Facebook.com/shahramshiva1
www.twitter.com/shahramshiva
www.instagram.com/shahramshiva
www.youtube.com/shahramshiva
www.pinterest.com/shahramshiva

Contact, Copyright Permissions, Queries and Bookings
info@rumi.net

Topics

When you dance the whole universe dances.

All the realms spun around you in endless celebration.

Your soul loses its grip.

Your body sheds its fatigue.

Hearing my hands clap and my drum beat,

You begin to whirl.

-- Rumi

Transformative Whirling
History of the Method

An Experience in Ecstasy

Whirling is for all of humanity and does not belong to any one part of the world, a certain religion or a spiritual sect. People from all countries and all faiths have been turning, spinning or whirling since the beginning of time.

When you watch children spin don't you envy their fun? Children everywhere love the freeing sense of spinning, and it doesn't matter what continent they are twirling on. Whirling belongs to all of humanity.

Back in 1995, I invented a unique new breakthrough technique that makes it possible for all to turn comfortably, competently, without any dizziness or discomfort. The beauty of my system and key to its success are in its simplicity.

Why Whirl

Whirling is as natural to us as walking. As mentioned above we have been whirling for thousands of years. Our universe manifests its energy through the spiral, hence as we whirl we harmonize with this energy; we tap into the core of our universe.

Whirling affects you on physical, mental, spiritual and psychological levels.
Whirling can instantly change your mood. It can brighten it and bring a smile to your face.

Whirling is a meditative movement and a form of meditation. Whirling can almost instantly create a state of meditation. I call it "active meditation" vs. the classic Buddha posture which I call "passive meditation." This active form of meditation helps center the body and the mind within a short few minutes.

Whirling is an ancient form of centering and meditation. It has been used in many spiritual cultures throughout the world. Through whirling we harmonize with the energy of the creation and form a more positive energy around us. Dervishes drop their black cloaks (a representative of their bodies) and begin to whirl as divine entities wearing all white. They believe that while they are whirling they are closest to being divine.

Whirling is a wonderful form of zero to low impact exercise. Whirling is also good for weight loss. Practicing whirling on regular basis will keep you lean, vibrant and full of energy.

Tapping Into the Core of the Universe

All matter in our universe is in a constant state of spinning, from subatomic particles to solar systems and galaxies. Every particle in our body and all that is around us are already spinning. Actually the Milky Way galaxy that our solar system is a part of is spinning in a spiral fashion as you read this.

My method is based on basic laws of physics and the common thread between all physical manifestations. This method is non-ritualistic by design. Students by following this proven method without any prior training can begin whirling immediately.

History of the Method

Since 1995, I have helped tens of thousands of people to whirl comfortably and competently. Some of my whirling students, including Deepak Chopra, teach this method in their workshops.

My guided group whirling has been featured on CNN, and I've taught it for many years at Kripalu Center, Omega Institute, NY Open Center among many other universities and institutions. I've worked with choreographers and stage directors for whirling shows. Also performed and have trained dancers to whirl at New York's Joyce and LaMama theaters. I also trained the actor Robert Downey Jr. to whirl in the movie Game 6.

I've so far successfully worked with groups as large as 400, although even larger groups can easily be guided. I envision stadiums filled with whirling enthusiasts, spinning in unison.

Recreating the Eye of a Tornado

In early '90s after having been whirling for a few years I discovered a curious connection between they way I was whirling, and the way the Earth rotates, a tornado spins and the solar system holds its proper order. I knew that all things in creation are in a state of perpetual whirling, from subatomic particles to galaxies. But then I realized that all things whirl/rotate/orbit/spin around an axis. This common thread is what my four-step method is about.

Just as the Earth turns around its axis, or the entire solar system orbits around the Sun, or a tornado spins around its eye, or the electrons circle around the protons, we can create an axis within our body to whirl around it. It takes only a few minutes to learn this method. The best thing about this method is that it works regardless of your age or your physical

training, and just like yoga you can set
your own pace.
Of course those who are in better
physical shape tend to spin faster. I have
seen some participants in my workshops
after just one try to whirl at an amazing
pace with much comfort, but it's not just
about the speed of rotation. I am happy to
have designed this quick method and to
be sharing it with you.

We whirl counter clockwise to uplift the
soul to the heavens. Some cultures
(Buddhist in particular) tend to keep the
option of whirling clockwise if they feel
the need to bring a more grounded
balance to their energy.

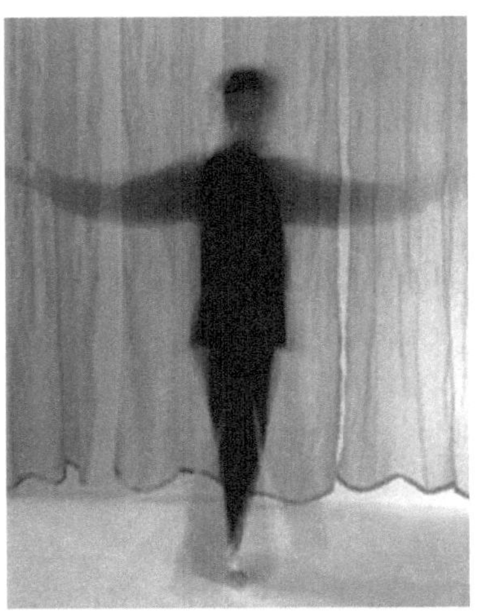

Shahram Shiva's Unique & Proven Four-Step Method to Whirling

The following four-step method has been field-tested in hundreds of workshops with tens of thousands of participants since the '90s.

Before you begin make sure that:
- The ground you are whirling on is stable and level.
- You are not whirling on small rugs, blankets or mats that can move under you.
- You are not wearing shoes.
- You are wearing socks on smooth surfaces, or are barefooted on carpets.
- You are not wearing glasses.
- You have ample room to move about freely in your space, and keep a radius of at least 10 feet around you free of any obstacles.
- You are trying this on an empty stomach.
- You will follow the instruction as stated. Do not attempt to improve them, or take shortcuts, you will not be successful.

- Do exactly as stated. Otherwise I recommend not attempting my method.

Step One: Stand

Everything in the universe is in a constant state of spinning and everything is perpetually turning around an axis. If you look at the above image (P63), you'll notice that I created an axis with my body that my arms turn around it. Just stand in a comfortable natural erect posture. Please turn counter clockwise or toward your heart or to the left and know that only one in every thousand tornadoes turn clockwise and the entire solar system including the Earth, rotate counter clockwise (there are a couple of planets that are exceptions due to collisions).

Step Two: Turn Around Your Left Foot

Just like a top that spins around a point, we will create this point by turning around the ball of our left foot. Please note that this is not Ballet and you do not need to actually turn around the ball of your foot constantly. The entire process is highly organic and very natural in approach. Therefore, turn around the ball of your left foot as you lower and lift your left heel to accommodate it. Your right leg propels you forward as your left foot continues the turn. Keep the distance between your feet shoulder width.

Step Three: The Eyes

Look Straight. Keep Your Head Level.
Have Soft Focus.
Let's get this out of the way first: if you
have dance training please do not "spot"
(spotting will work against turning and
you will not be able to whirl for long). As
you start to whirl try to have soft focus.
Don't to look at anything but maintain an
unfocused vision. Let the images in the
room pass you by without your visual
participation. If you wear prescription
glasses take them off before whirling. If
you look at objects as you whirl, you will
not be able to have a smooth turn, and
you will be forced to stop your whirling
after a few short spins. Please do not
look at your hand either as you turn.
Whirling is about freedom; we don't try to
leave this cage of a body to fall into
another cage of locking our gaze on our
hands as we whirl.

Finally, keep your head level. Don't look
up and don't look down. Look straight
with your head level through out the

whirling session until you are ready to come to a stop.

Step Four: How To Stop?

When you feel that it's time to stop, first slowdown your rotation or whirling speed and get as slow as you can. Just as you are about to come to a stop, look down and pick a stationary object on the floor. It could be lint, a chair, a cushion, a pattern on a carpet, or a stain on a wooden floor. Now stop, stand comfortably, keep looking down and lock your focus on that object.

Please do not remove your focus until the room has completely stopped turning around you. This step is most crucial to help you have a dizzy-free experience. Be patient and wait for the sense of spinning room to come to an absolute halt. Now you can feel free to move about. Congratulations, you have had your first whirling experience.

Here are a Few More Pointers

- As you start to turn, stretch your arms comfortably, not too stiff though and keep your right palm up to the heavens and your left palm down to the earth. You receive the energy of the creation with your right palm and transmit the same energy with your left palm. This way you become a conduit for the transmission of the energy of the creation. You harmonize with the energy of the universe.
- Remember to breathe. Breathe, and be as comfortable as you can while whirling. The more you whirl, the easier and more effortless it becomes.
- Put on a music that you think is appropriate and has a steady beat (although music with a specific beat is not necessary, certain classical music or jazz will also do fine).
- Remember to keep your axis solid at all times, it is your pillar that you are turning around, so keep it

steady, and please try not to be too stiff.

- The more you try whirling the easier it gets. After a few successful whirling sessions you can gradually loosen up on the method.
- The 4-Step Method is designed to offer you an instant access to whirling, however, once you get good at whirling you no longer need the method and you can experiment with moving your arms and turn it into a dance if you like.
- Enjoy yourself, and have fun with this. Just like Yoga, find your own pace and experiment with it as you go along.

Warning

- A slight dizziness is normal after your first few tries, since your body needs time to get used to this new sensation.
- If you can't follow my directions exactly as stated, do not attempt.
- If you don't have the discipline to maintain soft focus through out, do not attempt.
- If you don't have the discipline to keep your head level at all times, except to stop, do not attempt. You maintain your balance with glands behind your ears, when you move your head you disturb the balance.
- If you have certain physical injuries or challenges that might prevent you from following my method, do not attempt.
- If you have certain medical conditions that might prevent you from following my method, do not attempt.
- I am neither responsible nor liable for any harm or injury that might

occur to those who attempt to whirl or move about, whether they follow my method or not, and for any other reason whatsoever, at any time and any place.
- Try this at your own risk.

Exercise Disclaimer

The exercises provided above are for educational and entertainment purposes only, and is not to be interpreted as a recommendation for a specific treatment plan, product, or course of action. Exercise is not without its risks, and this or any other exercise program may result in injury. They include but are not limited to: risk of injury, aggravation of a pre-existing condition, or adverse effect of over-exertion such as muscle strain, abnormal blood pressure, fainting, disorders of heartbeat, and very rare instances of heart attack. To reduce the risk of injury, before beginning this or any exercise program, please consult a healthcare provider for appropriate

exercise prescription and safety
precautions. The exercise instruction and
advice presented are in no way intended
as a substitute for medical consultation.
The author disclaims any liability from
and in connection with this program. As
with any exercise program, if at any point
during your workout you begin to feel
faint, dizzy, or have physical discomfort,
you should stop immediately and consult
a physician.

All Rights Reserved

This unique 4-Step Method to Whirling
has been created, designed and invented
exclusively by Shahram Shiva and it is a
legally protected technique. Mr. Shiva
holds all rights to this groundbreaking
method. The method shall not be taught
by others without proper credit and rights
request. For the rights to use this method
please email info@rumi.net.

The Famed Whirling Dervishes of Turkey do not Represent Rumi, they Epitomize his Son

Rumi wasn't part of a cult, neither was he a Sufi nor called anyone his master. After Sham's passing he wasn't anyone's disciple nor did he care to form an organized sect and to govern and lead followers. When he famously whirled, he did it whenever and wherever he wanted. Not in a choreographed fashion, but in an ecstatic, freeform, wild and spontaneous way.

The rigidly choreographed style of whirling that the famed Whirling Dervishes of Turkey perform did not start with Rumi but with his eldest son Sultan Walad several years after his passing. When it was finally time for Sultan Walad to take charge of Rumi's family, he formed a spiritual sect to honor his father and styled a type of whirling choreography that we witness today. In his design he placed a figure to represent Rumi in the center of the room and had the whirling students turn around him, like planets orbiting a sun.

Whirling in reality is never that rigid, predictable or choreographed. Many whirling troops outside of Turkey, in countries such as Iran, India, Egypt and Syria perform whirling with intense amount of passion and imagination and never repeat the same arm gestures or even body movements.

I have been teaching my own unique method to whirling since 1995 and I've always followed Rumi's impassioned, true-to-self and creative freestyle method and cared little for the high-conformity routine of the Whirling Dervishes of Turkey.

Additional Tools for Students of Spirituality and Self-Empowerment

How to Manifest
Your Vision

The great visionary Charles Chaplin in his 1952 movie Limelight talks about the law of desire and tapping into the universal energy. He says, "Life is a desire. Desire is the theme of all life... Think of the power that's in the universe... And that's the same power within you. If you'd only have courage and the will to use it."

Most successful people use visualization techniques to help manifest their goals and there are of course multitudes of books on the topic as well. But self-help books typically don't produce results; otherwise half of the planet would be living their dreams.

The universal energy is all around us, within and without. Science tells us that we are in fact stardust. We are as much a part of this universal energy as the stars, planets and nature.

Although we are part of this cosmic play, unless we learn to quiet our minds from the constant chatter, distraction and noise and focus our mental vibrations through meditation, we won't be able to fully tap into the universal energy.

The ideal way to project or beam your mental desires onto the universe and to help manifest your vision is not to form it as a novel, or a short story, an email, or even a text message it's best to say it as a one- or two-word phrase (or send a single image formed in your mind). For example if your vision is to become a professional pastry chef, no need to clutter your beam with too much info, all you need to say is "pastry chef." The term chef in English denotes professional affiliation.

So, condense your wish to one or two words and then focus on it and project it. Here's another example. Since I live in LA, I'll make it about wanting to become an actress. If that's the case, don't clutter your thoughts with too many details, such as whom you want to direct you, or for you to star with. Just say to yourself "successful actress." Why not just "actress," because if you just project "actress" you may end up in a community theater in a small town somewhere. OK, now let's begin.

Preparation

- Don't try this if you feel sleepy or your mind isn't fully awake.
- Put aside about 20 minutes and find a quiet place.
- Make sure you aren't disturbed during this time.
- Sit upright either on a chair or on the floor.
- Make sure you are comfortable.
- Keep a little journal next to you, whether your computer, your phone that has been put on mute or pen and paper.

Meditation and Projection

- Start your meditation. Keep eyes closed and breath slowly.
- Focus on what makes you happy.
- Don't force or judge the wishes and don't place monetary limitation on them.
- Trust your instinct and sense which thought, profession or scenario makes you truly happy.
- Keep it simple. Use my one- or two-word projection technique.
- Think of the people around you who are negative and do not support your vision, then say to yourself "less." Meaning you want less people like that around.
- Then think of the people around you who support your vision, then say to yourself "more." From now on, keep it only positive.
- Place no limitation or judgment on your wishes.
- Now continue to repeat your vision internally as you breathe in and out with your eyes closed.

After The Session

- After your session, type or write your thoughts and the exact nature of your vision and how you feel about it.
- Then focus on your vision and think about it daily.
- Your new clear and uncluttered focus will bring in events, people or situations that will help with your vision.
- Soon you'll find ways to manifest your dream.

Finally

Remember it doesn't have to be an epic decision, so small gestures are OK too. Stay positive. It's important that you maintain your focus on what you want following your vision manifestation session. Make sure to repeat these sessions often or at least once a week.

Understanding Mystic
or Yogic Dreams

Those of us who dream regularly and remember our dreams assume that the rest of the world also remembers theirs. However, only a percentage of the public recalls them and many claim not to dream at all.

Spiritual beings typically remember their dreams and can distinguish them by type, since not all dreams have the same intensity or hold equal value.

I categorize dreams into 4 distinct types:

1. Normal Dreams

Most dreams, as researchers suggest, are normal brain activity and rehashing of the day's memories, events, anxiety and persistent thoughts. Almost all such dreams are rather ordinary and are easily forgotten.

2. Dreamland

Some of the more interesting dreams happen in a zone I call the Dreamland, which is similar to a vast and crowded holographic arena that causes interaction between multitudes of human beings who are dreaming at the same time. In this crowded zone there are also various entities, mostly malevolent, who prey on the psyche of the dreamers. Same as any large train station, the Dreamland has no filter into who can enter; hence it is accessible to all. But unlike a modern day station it has no security force. Therefore in Dreamland it's your essence against theirs. Wit against wit. Willpower against willpower.

Dreamland in many ways is like an immersive virtual reality game. Nothing in dreamland is as it appears. Since there are many shape-shifting malevolent entities active in Dreamland, the more aware and more evolved you are mentally and spiritually the better you'll do there. Because your emotions and desires are totally transparent there, entities can easily project themselves as someone that you love, respect or lust after. To enhance their illusion, they can also create temporary facades, maze, clothing, food or vehicles.

A simple rule of deciphering good vs. bad entities or benevolent vs. malevolent spirits is that a malevolent will always try to get close to you or force him/herself on you, touch you or trap you in a small space. A benevolent entity, on the other hand, will never come closer than 10 to 12 feet, will never crowd, startle or scare you. There are times that a benevolent spirit may want to get close to you, as to embrace you, but this happens out of mutual trust and understanding, and it's never sudden nor forced.

Dreamland can teach you to protect and defend yourself. This is also a good place to learn to sore and fly. There are various ways that you can turn around a negative situation in Dreamland. First rule is to become good at sensing that you are actually dreaming. Once you become aware that you are in Dreamland then you'll have the upper hand.

Here are a few instant giveaways that you are in Dreamland. Although you maybe surrounded by electronic devices, switches or be operating vehicles, none works as it should. If you are driving a car or riding a motorcycle, you'll find yourself have little control over the vehicle or that the steering and the brakes don't work or if you crash you sustain no injury. While using a computer or your phone, the screen would show gibberish or static content. Your clothing or lack thereof may change from one moment to the next without cause. Or, you'll find yourself running around in an endless maze of corridors where there is no escape.

You may not realize while you are dreaming that you have control over the situation. As soon as you have any inkling that you are in Dreamland the gig is up and the advantage is now yours. At this time you can choose to fight back and break apart the maze or wake yourself up. If you choose to fight back you can summon a weapon. And you don't have to have full mastery of that weapon in real life to put it to good use. Like a video game, the Dreamland grants you temporary know-how into using that weapon. Remember nothing is real in Dreamland it's all projections; so don't feel bad about vaporizing a few of the bad guys. When it comes down to it, Dreamland is only a sophisticated mental hologram meant to train and strengthen you, make you learn to function outside your body and help you on your path to higher levels of soul evolution.

3. Mystic Dreams

Intense spiritual and transformational dreams are the playground of the benevolent spirits and ascended masters. Mystic Dreams are the rare transmission dreams. They normally happen early in the morning (around 4) and are vivid, in full color and very memorable. They may involve intense lights, colors, sights, sounds, aromas and music. Depending on the intensity of the transmission, you maybe half awake with your eyes and mouth open or full sleep but in either case your body will feel paralyzed as to expedite the process of the transference.

These dreams normally include a transmission or a teaching by a benevolent spirit or spirits and in most cases involve visual cues, icons, animal spirits, sounds, smells or direct verbal teachings and transference of information. You will not only remember such dreams, there is a good chance that you'll never forget them.

4. Dreams of Animal Spirits

There is a less intense version of Mystic Dreams, which involves animal spirits. In such dreams information, mostly about your near future, are transmitted by seeing specific animals in action (horses, bears, large cats, snakes, dogs, birds and so on).

It's important to try to remember not only the species but what the animal is doing in your dream. For example if it's a large cat, is it a lion, tiger or a panther. Is it docile and friendly or trying to attack you. If you dream of a horse, pay attention whether it's white, black or brown. But most importantly try to register and remember what you were thinking the moment that you saw that animal. That's your real clue for the meaning of that particular animal spirit dream.

There are many online websites that cater to dream interpretation, however these sites offer wildly diverse information. You may want to read a few such websites and then create your own version of the interpretation based on what makes sense the most to you. Don't forget it all begins and ends with you.

Happy Dreaming!

Soul Evolution Principal:
The Four Stages

Rumi's most famous quote in English is his promise to take you to a place that is "beyond" right and wrong, good and bad. A place well beyond religion and blind faith. I call Rumi's highest stage of soul evolution "the Beyond." It is the ultimate attainment of a spiritual seeker while still in the body.

Change, expansion and evolution are the reality of the physical universe. Our own planet has undergone near five billion years of evolution. However, we don't just evolve physically or as species, we also evolve mentally and conscientiously. Through reincarnation and maintaining an open mind our souls can also evolve and grow with no limit.

We are on a very long journey of the soul, however we can't move forward on this endless path without an open and free mind. As soon as we close our minds, because of religious dogma, fundamentalism, orthodoxy, misguided sense of spiritual elitism, or an enslaved sense of self (a mind that is enslaved to a guru, a sect, a god or deity) we stop evolving.

I have categorized my humanity's Soul Evolution Principal in 4 stages. Of course, a lower level mind doesn't know about the other steps. For example, while you are in Level 2 (religion), even if you read about the Level 4, chances are you would simply ignore it or consider it "crazy." However, a higher-level mind certainly is aware of the other 3 steps as it has been there before. I have seen on my Facebook page rather violent reaction from people in Levels 2 or 3 when they read about my Soul Evolution Principal, because it challenges their belief system.

Humanity's Soul Evolution Principal

Level 1 — The Animal or Primitive Mind

Those at Level 1 are only concerned with survival, physicality and reproduction. They aren't interested in higher spiritual aspiration, which is a carryover from their mostly new incarnation from the animal world. Almost all animals' main focus is work (food, survival, shelter) and reproduction. Hence the mind at this level stays the course.

Level 2 — Religion

Filled with dogma and fear of punishment, it introduces basically what is soul slavery. Religions of the world program the followers to worship invisible beings and deities and surrender notion of self. Some religions openly refer to their followers as "sheep." However, religion also brings about a vague concept of higher thinking and it introduces the principal of a divine soul. Even though it also invents the incredibly dark term "eternal damnation." Due to very strong programming and the closed minds of the followers, most souls will not be able to ascent beyond this level. In fact Level 2 dwellers are routinely quite fanatical about clinging to their religion.

Level 3 — Spirituality 101

As a progressive soul evolves it sees through and naturally sheds the simplistic mind and soul control tactics used in religion. Many souls looking for answers outside of religion are drawn to Eastern-style spirituality or what is commonly called yoga or yogic teachings.

Due to strong programming that also exists in basic spirituality the seeker wrongly considers spirituality to be the ultimate truth (a fanatical pattern carried over from Level 2) and falls into another mind trap. Spirituality 101 certainly is more evolved than religion, as it introduces more light into the teachings.

However, as religion may contain only five percent truth, the Spirituality 101 increases that dose to about 25 percent.

Spirituality 101 is only another step in our soul evolution and it shouldn't be considered to be the final step. Spirituality 101 is also dogmatic and tries to control people through fear. Whether it's fear of bad karma or fear of regression or fear of being disliked by the guru or by countless deities.

Many spiritual sects maintain the concept of soul slavery and promote slave mentality and worship. The followers are trained to use deities and gurus names as mantras and repeat their names with every breath, at all times or chant their names out loud for days on end. They also demand total surrender and minimize the affect of the mind and logic to keep their followers small and dependent.

The Spirituality 101 world is filled with agenda-driven men and women who prey on innocent and naive people. This, in some ways, is even tougher to evolve out of than religion. Most people will be stuck at this level for a long time since it involves even deeper programming.

Level 4 — The Beyond

Rumi calls my Level 4 the Beyond, it is a place beyond right or wrong, good or bad and dark or light. Once you understand and truly inhabit your soul's worth, your true origin, your infinite path and ultimate destination, you'll gradually evolve beyond the basic spirituality as well. Your soul reaches adulthood and it then can become independent. All the past shenanigans and con artistry fade away. The thoughts of soul slavery go away. New revelations are revealed each day.

You transform from a slaved-soul to an empowered-soul. You change from a dependent-spirit to a self-guided entity.

The process of Soul Evolution is about maturity of the soul and its readiness for ascension off this dark planet.

You transform from that of a child soul needing boundaries and reward and punishment control methods to a mature soul that no longer requires any limitations.

The Beyond is where your soul journey starts actually. Up until now you have just been in training. You need strength of the soul, strong sense of self and acceptance of the notion of self-love. Only progressive souls with infinite thirst for the truth and clear, open minds can get to this point. Dogma and hypocrisy don't have a place here. The Beyond is the goal of all committed spiritual seekers.

A true Lover doesn't follow any one
religion,
be sure of that.
Since in the religion of Love,
there is no irreverence or faith.

Personal Gratitude

Rumi is a fire-breather. Masters like Rumi don't incarnate on this planet to tell you to smell the roses, they demand transformation. For beings like Rumi it's all about the burning, the fire and being cooked or being prepped for a higher purpose and elevated experiences free from all systems of control.

Having lived with Rumi and sharing his work with the world every day for the past 30 years has been one of my greatest pleasures and highest honors.

To have Rumi and Shams as mentors offer some of the most genuine and most powerful personal growth and soul evolution experiences at anytime in our collective history. It has also been a journey free from hypocrisy and shenanigans so rampant in all religious and spiritual circles.

Oh friend, always face the light as you move constantly forward and upward. Rise above fear. Maintain an open mind.

Don't fall victim to blind faith. Don't be afraid of the dark side. You are love and loved!

About Shahram Shiva

Shahram Shiva is an author, writer, poet, recording artist and award-winning translator and scholar of Rumi.

He is the founder of Rumi Network and one of the original translators and popularizers of Rumi. Shahram Shiva's Rumi interpretations are quoted and referred to in about 300 books in English and other languages.

He is a teacher of advanced spirituality (aka ascension). He is known for rich and entrancing concerts and performances, captivating talks and powerful experiential workshops.

Shahram Shiva's teachings are on the future of spirituality, consciousness expansion, vision manifestation, enlightenment, ascension and self-realization.

Shahram Shiva's latest books are 12 Secret Laws of Self-Realization and Rumi's Untold Story. Love Evolve is his last album to date.

Shahram Shiva's Bibliography

- 12 Secret Laws of Self-Realization: A Guide to Enlightenment and Ascension by a Modern Mystic. Rumi Network.

- Rumi's Untold Story: From 30-Year Research. Rumi Network.

- Transformative Whirling: Shahram Shiva's Unique & Proven 4-Step Method to Whirling. Rumi Network.

- Rumi, Thief of Sleep: Quatrains from the Persian. Foreword by Deepak Chopra. Hohm Press.

- Hush, Don't Say Anything to God: Passionate Poems of Rumi. Jain Publishing.

- Rending the Veil: Literal and Poetic Translations of Rumi. Hohm Press. (Recipient of the Benjamin Franklin Award)

- A Garden Beyond Paradise: The Mystical Poetry of Rumi. With Jonathan Star. Bantam Books (Random House).

Shahram Shiva's Discography

- Love Evolve, a collection of 10 songs. A mix of Rumi poetry set to music, and original songs with lyrics by Shahram Shiva. Produced by the GRAMMY Award-winner Danny Blume and Shahram Shiva.

- Rumi: Lovedrunk (Remastered), 2012 Release. A remastered release with enhanced sound and new cover design. A collection of 10 songs with lyrics based on Rumi poems, as translated and interpreted by Shahram Shiva. Produced by Olivier Glissant and Shahram Shiva.

- Rumi: Lovedrunk, a collection of 10 songs with lyrics based on Rumi poems, as translated and interpreted by Shahram Shiva. Produced by Olivier Glissant and Shahram Shiva.